Challenged

12

Near Death

Experience 1

Stay in Shape to Survive
Stroke

Eliahu Farkas

Dedication

Thank you Dror, Amos, Noa, Chen, Muli, and Advah for suffering my foibles, and for coming to the rescue whenever I dare catastrophe.

I dedicate this story to you.

Privileged to love you,
Eliahu Farkas

Forward

We meet surprises at every turn of our lives. Some good, some bad. Some comical, some sad. Some life-enriching, some life-threatening.

What do we learn from all our experiences?

This short story shares a real life-threatening event in the author's life. It could have ended badly—in death. One or more people could have lost their lives. Luckily, we didn't. We lived to tell the tale. We lived to grow and strive and smile.

Woven between the breath holding-lines of this suspense story, you will find universal life-lessons. You might even want to practice them...even share with your family and friends.

Enjoy, practice, and share.

Eliahu Farkas

Contents

Near Death

Almost over
Promise
Revived

Almost Over

Enjoying our usual early morning bike ride.

Just finished racing each other to Namal, on our bikes: Sun on his cyclocross and me on my road-bike. Both, top brands, as befits sworn cyclers. We made good time. Near our record time. We're having our reward coffee at the marina, watching the seagulls diving for fish, with the rising sun at our backs. We're schmoozing, discussing work issues and plans.

Sun snaps his fingers at me:

"Did you hear what I just said?"

"Yes," I nod. But I don't really remember what he said only a minute ago. I'm pretending.

As usual, Sun is antsy, in a hurry to beat the traffic into the office. He hustles me back onto the bike. I get on it as usual and start pedaling. After covering barely one kilometers, Sun overtakes me, jumps off his bike, steps in front of my bike, and grabs it by the handlebars.

"Get off the bike!" he screams at me.

I'm confused. I can't quite make out what he's saying.

Sun grabs me by the shoulders and sits me down on the nearest bench, facing the sea. He jabbers at me, but I can't make out what he's saying. He grabs his cell-phone and dials my wife, Sparrow.

"Something is wrong with Elku!" he yells into the mouthpiece.

"Sparrow wants to speak to you," Sun yells at me, shoving the cell phone in my hand and pushing it to my ear.

I hear a woman's voice, but can't make out what she's saying. I barely make out her saying: "Let me speak to Sun!"

I hand the phone back to Sun, who's very agitated. He speaks excitedly to my wife. I hear the word "ambulance." I also hear something about calling my children, and about some hospital. Vaguely, I recognized the hospital name. It was the nearest one.

He then turns to me and says:

"Sparrow is calling for an ambulance. She's also going to ask her friend, Mir, to alert her son Hag, a doctor at the hospital."

I barely make out meaning of Sun's words, and try to argue. But no matter how many times I repeat myself, Sun doesn't seem to understand what I'm saying. I'm frustrated, but cloudy and fuzzy.

Some time passed. I don't remember how much. Suddenly, there is a stranger in front of me. He seems to be dressed in white. He bends over and puts his face up close to mine. I can barely make out his features. He asks:

"What's your name?"

I answer "Elku," but he doesn't seem to understand.

I speak more slowly, enunciating carefully "E L K U!" But the man in white refuses to understand.

He puts up his hand, spreading his fingers apart, and asks: "How many fingers?"

I answer "five."

The man in white repeats the question: "How many fingers?"

Again, I answer: "Five, damn it!"

I'm annoyed he doesn't understand me. I'm very frustrated, and getting angry. I take my time, enunciating slowly, carefully, and emphatically: "F I V E!"

But still, the man in white refuses to understand what I'm saying. I'm frustrated. I'm not getting through to them.

But I'm fading. I can't make out what the man in white is saying. I think he's telling Sun and the other man in white "we'll have to rush him to the hospital!"

I feel I'm being trundled along over some rough surfaces. I hear engine noise, sirens, and bumps. And then, I pass out.

The next thing I remember is lying on a stretcher on top of a gurney. There are other vehicles around. Bustle of activity, but quiet. I'm surrounded by many people. I hear a commotion around me, but can't see any of the people, except a white-clad young woman to my left. I tilt my head to the left, trying to make out her features. I can't. I can barely make out that she's barking orders at others surrounding me, whom I can't see. Sounds like something about injections.

I hear garbled speech: "inject ... lift him ... push ... call ahead ... move him..."

I don't remember being rushed into the hospital building. I don't remember the next three days. I was out cold. No pain. No sensations. No dreams.

Promise

My loved ones were terrified. They were sure I was leaving them...

It was the only time anyone saw my dearest Sparrow crying. She was terrified. She thought she was going to lose me. A young doctor tried to calm her.

"He'll make it through," he promised.

Revived

The young doctor kept his promise. We thanked him long after, when we met him at the same hospital and I was no longer bed-bound.

I survived to tell and write about it. Checked out of the hospital some time afterwards; resumed normal life; resumed biking again; carried on.

You too can persist. Stay in shape to survive health mishaps. Never give up.

What Next?

Resume living
Charge forward
Stay in shape to stay alive

"What do you do after a major episode?" you ask.

Resume Living
Resume where you paused. Regard your episode as a passing event. But do not disregard its lessons. Avoid repeating the mistakes you made in the past. Hone your habits to include both, mind building and body building activities.

Read books that stimulate your imagination and broaden your horizons. Read story books, as well as drama, history, science, technology...the list goes on. Nothing is off the menu. Everything you read will stimulate your mind, opening new questions and horizons. Dare, try your hand at writing down your own thoughts.

Build your body by returning to your childhood. Remember how you enjoyed running, skipping, climbing, chasing a ball, riding bikes, swimming, diving. You must have had many other enjoyable activities that made you smile. Why don't you revisit them? Don't say "I'm too old for this..."

You're never too old to have fun, gallivanting about and being mischievous. Just do it! Your fitness and skills will return without you noticing. In no time at all, you'll find yourself smiling and waiting restlessly for the next opportunity to go out and play.

Do NOT become sedentary!

Charge Forward
Broaden your horizons. Take on new challenges. Lead.

Now is the best time to try something new. It may be a hobby, volunteer activities, or going back to school. Certainly, not a time for slouching around doing nothing.

Stay in Shape to Stay Alive

Although I learned the importance of staying fit, exercising regularly, and having fun, my near-death episode reinforced those precepts. So long as you make physical activity a part of your routine, on a regular basis, it doesn't matter. Do what you enjoy most, but do not take to extreme. Day-on, day-off, is generally recommended for most people.

Here are some pros and cons for some popular sports. The choice is yours. Put the emphasis on smiling.

"Don't all sports make you smile, light up your eyes, bond you to others?" you ask.

Of-course there are. But most are either logistically complex, damage one or another part of your body, or need time set-asides.

Take swimming. You need a pool. Unfortunately, for most of us, pools are not within walking distance. When you want to swim, you need to prepare a bag of equipment, travel to the pool, change into swimming trunks, shower after the swim, dress, and commute back.

Most ball sports, such as tennis, require a court. Again, must reserve a court in advance, can use the court only for the allotted time, schlep to a neighborhood that has the required facilities, dress, shower. After we're done, we have to go through the same steps again, in reverse order, consuming even more time.

Boating requires a lake, ocean, boats, and associated paraphernalia, such as special clothing and equipment, as well as navigation and safety gear. Usually, very expensive. There's always something more you need or broken equipment that needs replacing. Getting out there and returning usually consumes more time than the boating activity itself.

"What remains within reach of normal mortals?" you ask frustratingly.

"Jogging?" you wonder.

Although popular, jogging has hidden penalties that crop up years later.

As any orthopedic surgeon will tell you: "Jogging is harmful to your joints musculature, and bones!

Jogging grinds your spine, joints, bones, and the cartilage between them—all non-renewable and painful upon loss. Nothing much hurts more than bone rubbing against bone, or a stiff back—common in both younger and older people. Unfortunately, jogging harms both women and men. We all endure the penalty of misusing our bodies while running. Many joggers must desist because of pain and permanent damages: spinal damage, flattened/torn cartilages, hair-line bone cracks, torn muscles. The list goes on.

 "Walking then?" you attempt feebly.

Yes, walking is good. But it's tediously, boringly monotonous. You don't cover much ground. The view stays the same. Moreover, if carried to extreme, walking may also result in some of the harms incurred from jogging.

"Prefer biking," say the experts.

Why?

Biking hardly suffers from the shortcomings of jogging or walking. It spreads your weight over three points: your legs, your perineum (the bony inciteable region between the pubic arch and the tail bone), and your arms. Better still, as you become skilled, you can modulate each of these three areas, shifting weight and strain minutely for maximum comfort and pleasure. As you gain experience and fitness, you'll learn to stand, soaking up the bumps with your leg muscles, resting the other parts of your body, and gaining better control of your bike.

Few activities put a smile on your face as bicycling. Your eyes will light up, and you won't be able to wipe the smirk off your face for hours—during and after your bike ride. Careening on two wheels takes you back to your childhood, having fun churning your legs, twisting, turning, daring, and showing off. You might even be mischievous, as when you were a kid. You might lift the front wheel in the air, riding only on one wheel. You might jump hurdles. You never know where that rediscovered mischievousness might take you.

Biking saved my life—not once, twice!

First time I was saved by biking was when I was in mid-ocean kayaking, on the verge of drowning. The fitness I developed from churning the pedals gave me the strength and stamina to paddle my kayak back to safety. After saving my friend's life, after he capsized in mid-ocean, I was exhausted and sea-sick. If I weren't fit, both my friend and I would have died far out at sea.

The second time cycling saved my life was when I suffered a stroke. Most people who suffer a stroke, are paralyzed in parts of their bodies and may lose speech and other brain-dependent functions. I didn't suffer these extreme outcomes because, as brain scans showed, the blood vessels in my brain were widened beyond normal. That's why the blockage of blood flow was only partial, minimizing the dire consequences of typical strokes.

Important as physical health is, mental and spiritual health are even more important. Without them there is no cheer and no motivation in your life. Riding puts a smile on your face. It lights up your eyes. It bonds you to others. No logistical hassles. Just roll your bike out the front door, mount it, and pedal away.

Few other activities will exercise your balance and reflexes as safely and as well as bicycling. If that's not reason enough, biking is accessible. You don't need to travel to a special facility or location. Right outside your front door, on any day at any time, is the perfect place to both start and finish. You can do nature and sight-seeing on special occasions.

Biking is social. Do it with your mate, children, grandchildren, relations, friends, riding clubs...

Great way to bond with those you cherish.

Great way stay healthy.

Great way to keep smiling.

Recommended Biking Regime

Ride Safe

Don't overdo it!

Drink, drink, drink

Salt balance

Protect your skin

Day on—day off

Warm up—cool off

Change Scenery

Don't push—pull damn it!

Ride hard—ride easy

Vary riding styles

Smile smile smile!

Ride Safe
First and foremost, **RIDE SAFE!**

Do not attempt anything beyond your skill level.

Take every precaution to avoid harm or accidents—both, to yourself or to others.

Avoid competing with traffic or with pedestrians. Always prefer reserved bicycle paths or open spaces.

Don't Overdo it!
Don't attempt anything beyond your skill or endurance levels. Start slowly and improve your skill.

Avoid dangerous maneuvers or risky terrain until you acquire and practice the necessary skills. It's always a good idea to be accompanied by a skilled mentor who will also help protect you from harm as you gradually try more daring maneuvers.

Lengthen the amount of time on the bike, and the distance covered gradually, as your fitness improves.

Drink, Drink, Drink
Don't forget to hydrate. Keep in mind that while riding you lose a lot of liquids through sweat and through breathing. It's even worse on hot days. However, be careful not to drink too much because overhydration can dilute the salt balance in your body to dangerously low levels.

Salt Balance
Your body needs salt for proper operation of the nervous system and other organs in your body.

Most if not all energy bars contain some salt, to maintain correct ion balance. If in doubt, or if you don't use energy bars, put a tiny bit of salt in your water or in your home-made snacks. My practice is to wet the tip of my finger, dip it in a bit of table salt, and lick.

Don't overdo this either. If in doubt, to avoid creating new health problems, consult with your doctor.

Protect your Skin

You can help reduce loss of liquids by wearing long sleeved shirts and long trousers. Commercially available riding clothes are very good at evaporating excess perspiration to keep your body cool and maintain a good level of hydration. Long sleeves and trousers are also the best protection against sunburn.

Just ask Bedouins why they wear long clothes in the 'heat furnace' of the cloudless desert. Centuries of experience taught them that it's better to protect their skin with dark, long woolen clothes, then expose it searing sun.

Day On—Day Off

The opposite of *too little* is *too much*.

If you've not ridden at all, don't go overboard, overdoing it with excessive time on your bike.

Rule No. 1—Start Gradually:

Build up your stamina gradually. Half an hour per ride should be more than enough at the beginning. Also, prefer flat ground with no climbs or descents.

As you lengthen the time on the saddle, your body will build up to meet the challenge.

Rule No. 2—Day On-Day Off:
Avoid riding on consecutive days. You need to give your body a chance to replenish torn muscle fibers, and build new muscle tissue.

Warm Up—Cool Off

Every time you go riding, avoid shocking your body by immediately charging away at full speed. If you've ever watched professional bike riders, you'll see them spending quite a long time pedaling on rollers or treadmills in advance of the actual race. They're doing that to warm up in advance of the actual ride.

If you don't have rollers or a treadmill, simply ride gently, on an easy gear, for the first one to three kilometers of your ride. Warm your legs and tune your lungs and heart before you go full blast.

Tip: you might prefer rollers over treadmills because:

Cost
Rollers should be less expensive to buy.

Space
Rollers may be more compact and easier to stow away when not in use.

Bother
Rollers do not require removing your bike's rear wheel, setting it up on the treadmill, then unhooking from the treadmill, and putting the wheel back on the bike. With

rollers on the other hand, you simply get on to warm up and get off to set out riding.

Improve your Balance

Whereas on a treadmill, your bike is clamped firmly in place, not so on rollers. Your bike can move sideways from side to side as you pedal. Although it'll feel scary at first, it'll actually help you learn not to yaw from side to side as you pedal. Practicing on rollers will teach your body to maintain straight course, directing your energy into moving forward and not side-to-side.

Yes, there's a good chance you'll lose your balance on rollers at first. We recommend you ask a friend to steady you or do it in a doorway to prevent falling off. You should get the hang of it pretty quickly. Just let your body do its thing.

Change Scenery

Riding in the same places time and time again can get boring. Chose new places. Find scenic routes. Ride on the waterfront. Ride in the woods. Find new places you've never ridden before.

It's a good idea to plan in advance, seeking routes and maps for your next ride. There's plenty to choose from in the internet and other sources. You may ride with a group whose leaders are resourceful and find interesting new places for each ride.

Don't Push—Pull Damn It

The muscles under your thigh, back, are stronger and better pivoted than those on top of your thigh, front. Same as the muscles in front of your arm being stronger than those in the back.

Most bike riders rely on the muscles on top of their thighs, simply because that's how they were taught as children, before they learned to cleat their feet to the pedals.

Learn to ride with cleats, connecting your feet to the pedals. Then, train yourself to pull the pedals rather than push them.

Better still, learn to spin the pedals—but that's for advanced training, taught elsewhere.

Ride Hard—Ride Easy

Careful how you build your stamina and endurance. Don't drive your body too hard. Tip: ride hard, then ride easy. You can do it in each ride, riding out hard, returning gently. Or vary on alternate riding days: riding hard one day and easy on another.

Vary Riding Styles

There are numerous riding styles, and newer ones invented all the time. Most of us become accustomed to one style of riding and one type of bike. That's a shame, because we humans like variety.

You can putter around your neighborhood, do long road rides, cross-country rides, technical mountain rides, scary daredevil rides...the list is as long as our inventiveness and imagination.

Variety is the spice of life. Try new riding styles, fresh locations and scenery, different bike types, and riding with different people.

Smile Smile Smile
And most important of all: do not wipe that smile off your face. Become that young kid again, gleeful and unfettered. Enjoy thinking about the upcoming ride. Imagine the route in your mind while lying in bed, and plan for it.

Smile, smile, smile!